6 Green Smoothie Recipes

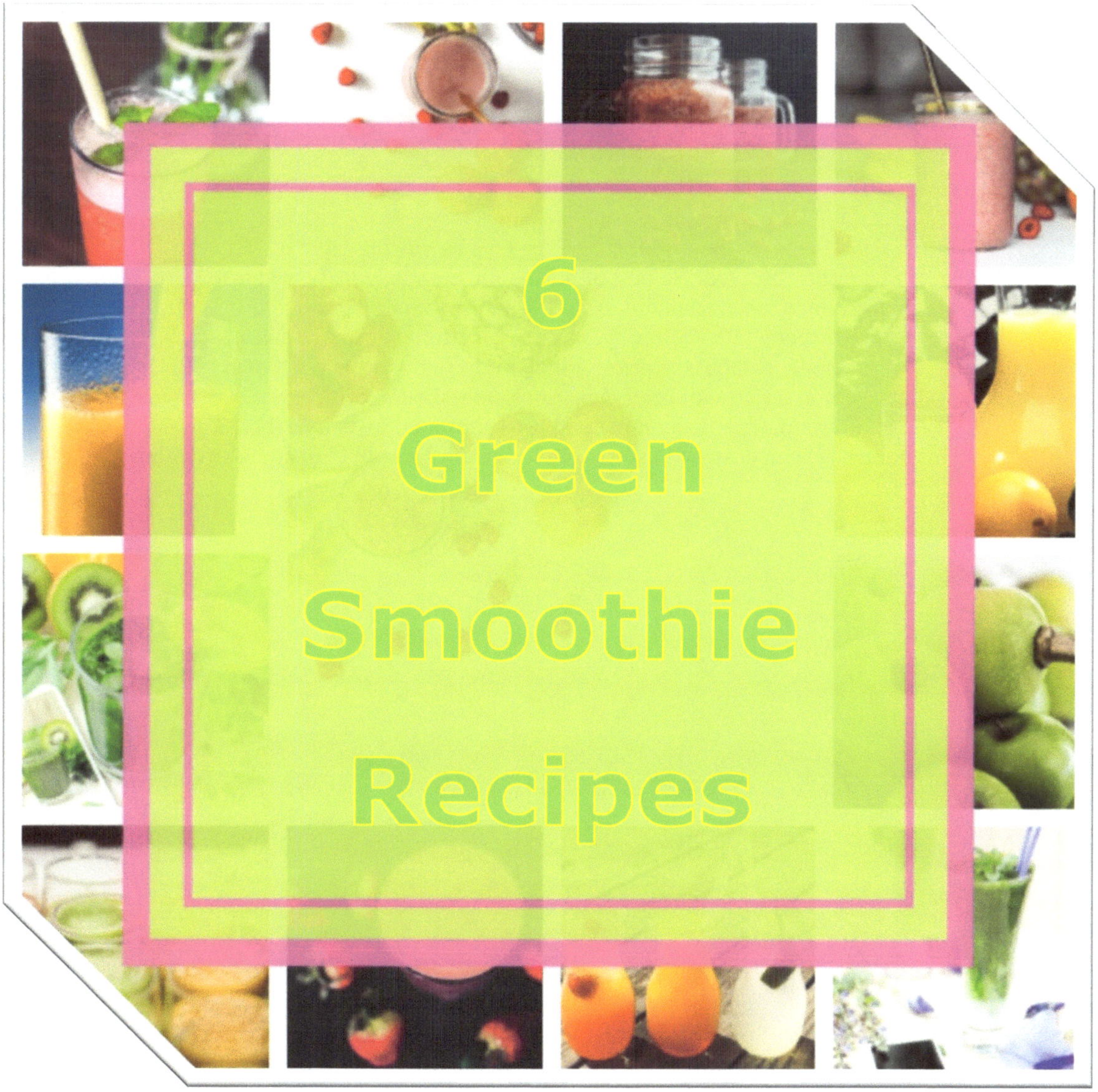

These recipes are dedicated
to you - my friends
who want to get health
by drink green smoothies.

Thank you!

How to Make Smoothie?

Just blend
and/or blend again
to make it smoothest.
You may add some water
and/or ice cubes as needed
than enjoy it immediately.

Green Smoothie Recipes

1. Green Dream Smoothie
2. Kale Smoothie
3. Spinach Smoothie
4. Collard Green Smoothie
5. Celery Smoothie
6. Grapes Smoothie

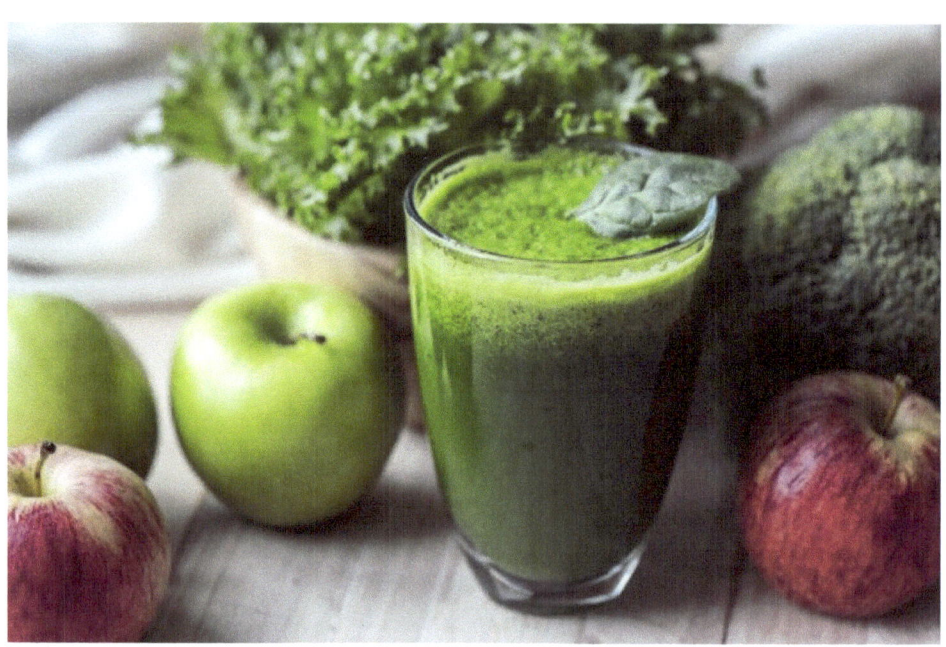

6

Green

Smoothie

Recipes

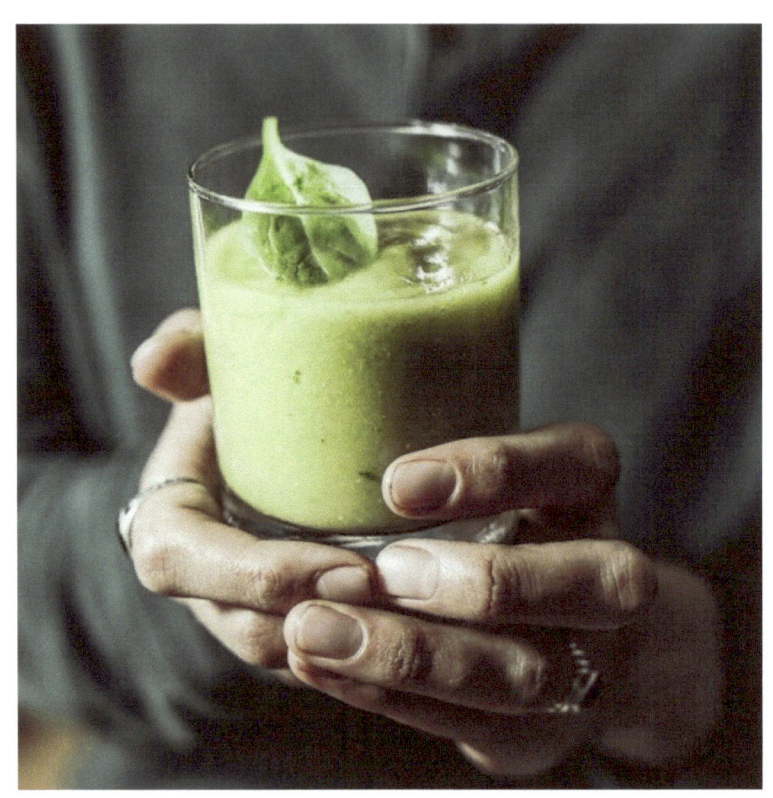

There are smoothies.
There are green smoothies.
Which one would you choose?

I would prefer green smoothies since they are a fusion of vegetables and fruits and you get both the sides!

Sneaking green vegetables in your food can not systematically make you happy, but you can thoroughly consume green smoothies to get that much necessary nutrition from the vegetables you often evade.

Here are 6 Green Smoothie Recipes for you.

1. Green Dream Smoothie

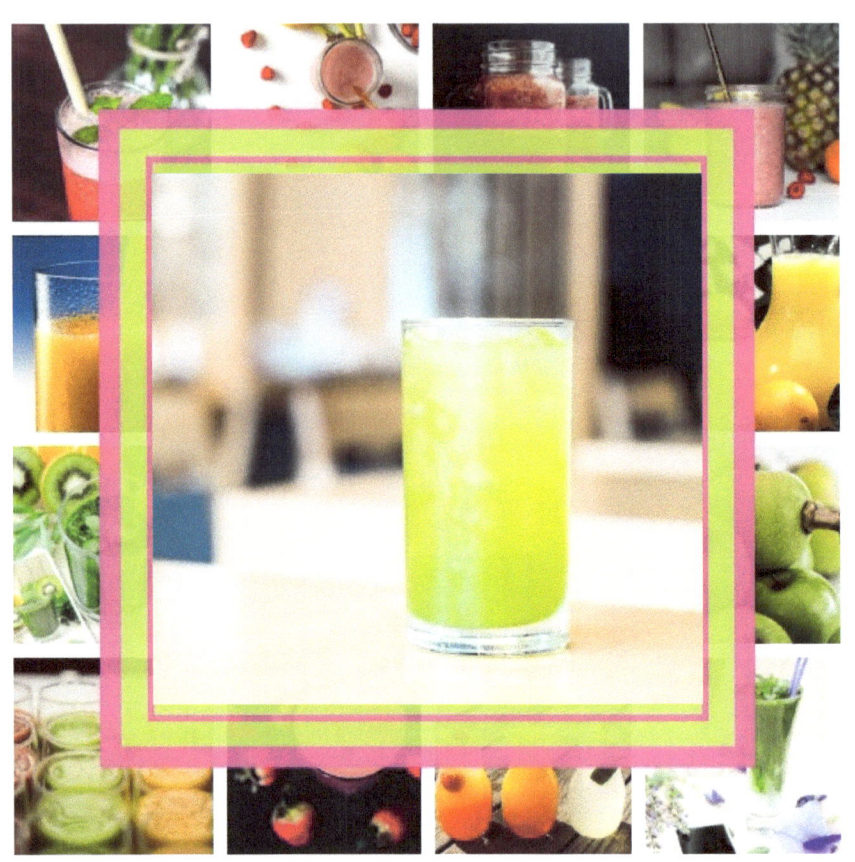

Baby Spinach 1.5 cups
Frozen Mango 1 cup
Banana 1 cup
Juice of 1 lemon

2. Kale Smoothie

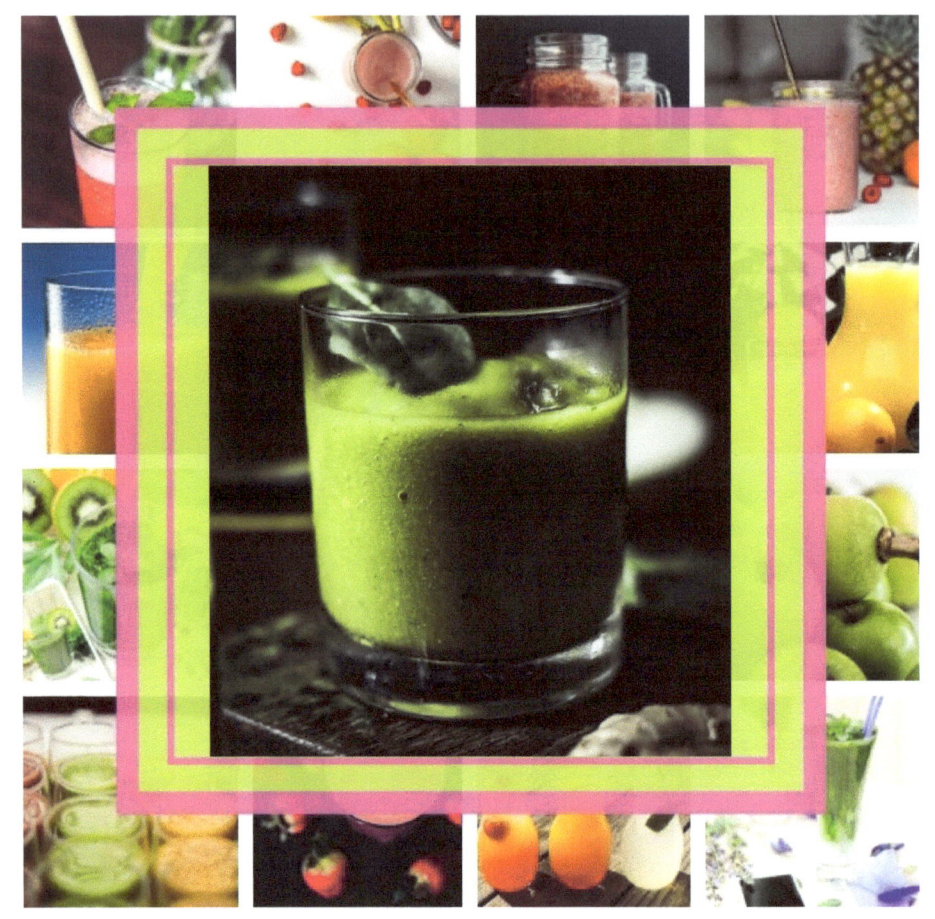

Kale 1/2 cup
Almond milk 1 cup
Banana 1 whole

3. Spinach Smoothie

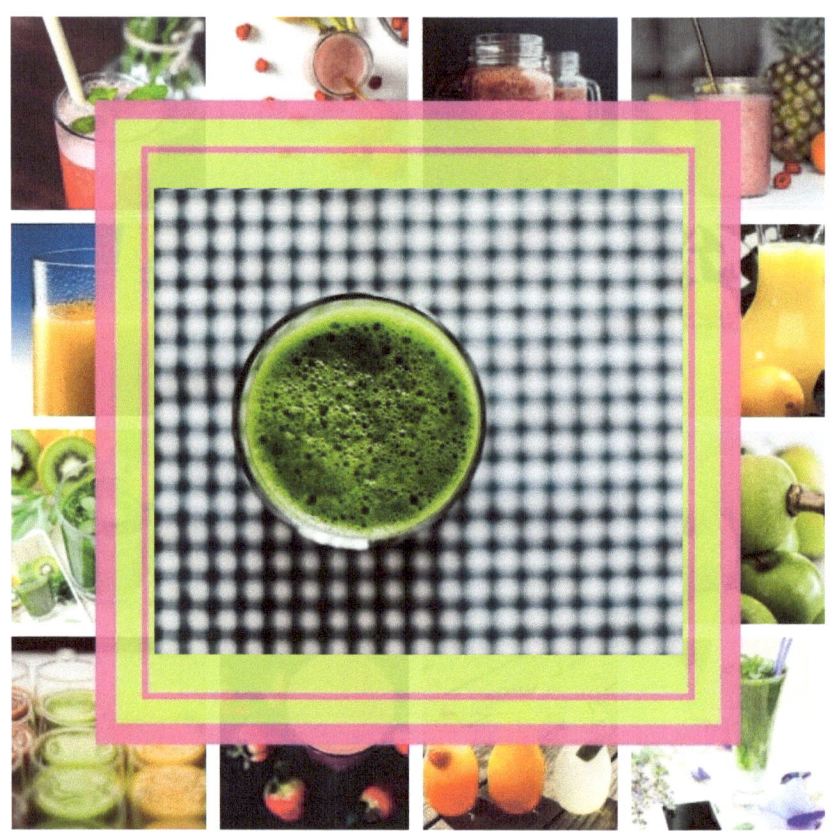

Spinach 1/2 cup
Yogurt 1 cup
Frozen Raspberry 1 cup

4. Collard Green Smoothie

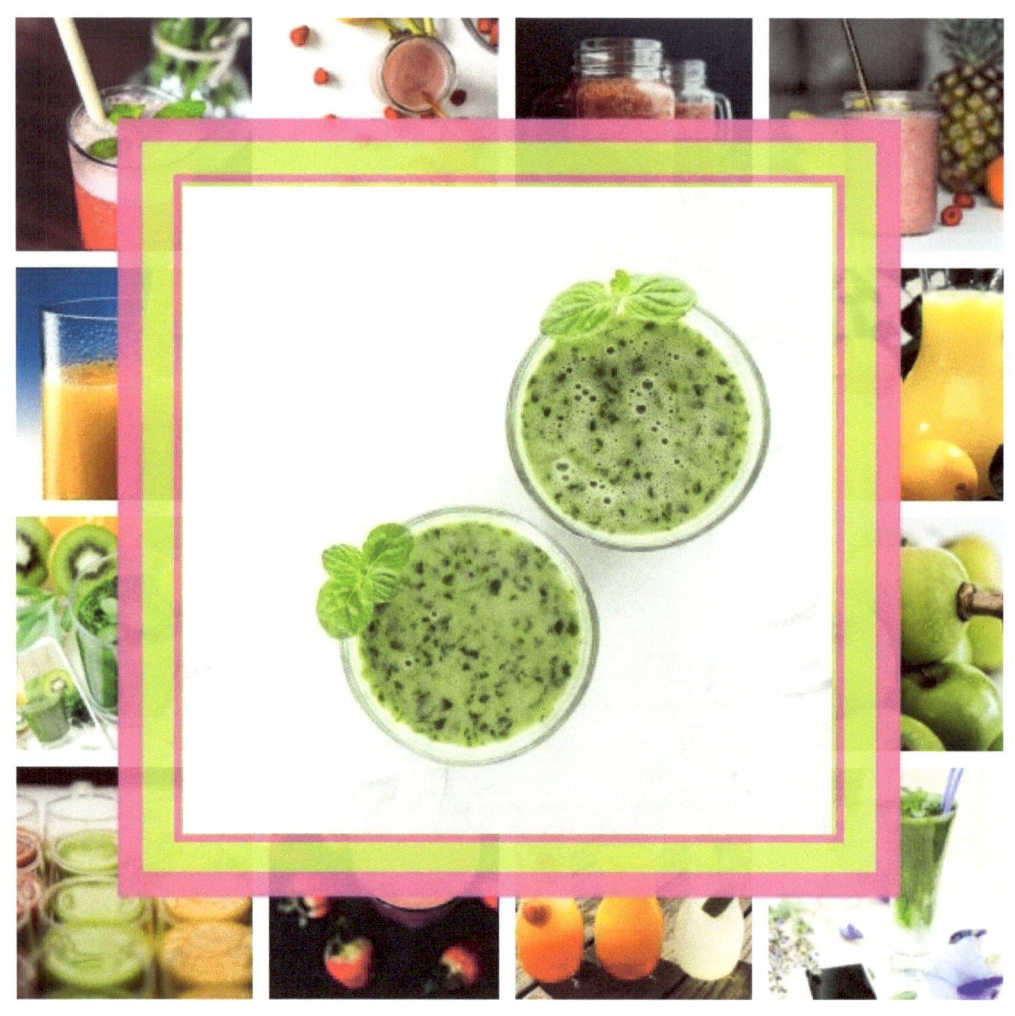

Collard Greens 1/2 cup
Lime juice 2 tablespoons
Apples 2 cups

5. Celery Smoothie

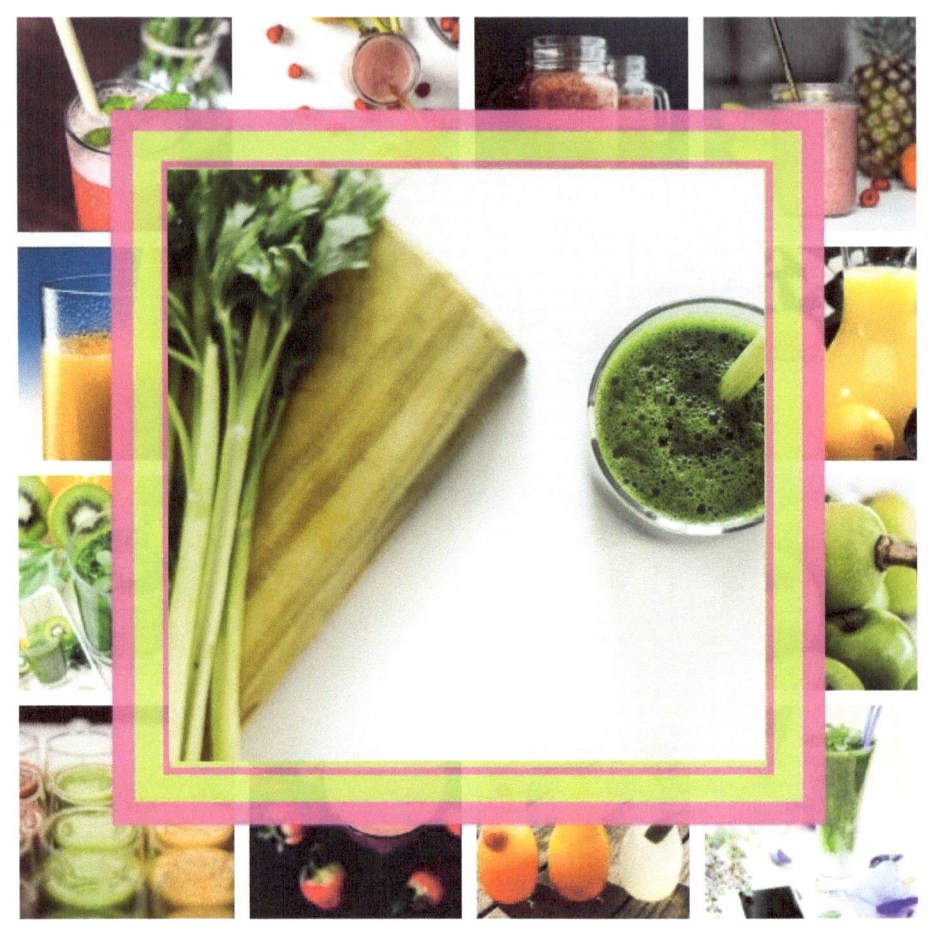

Celery 1/2 cup
Coconut water 1 cup
Pineapple 2 cups diced

6. Grapes Smoothie

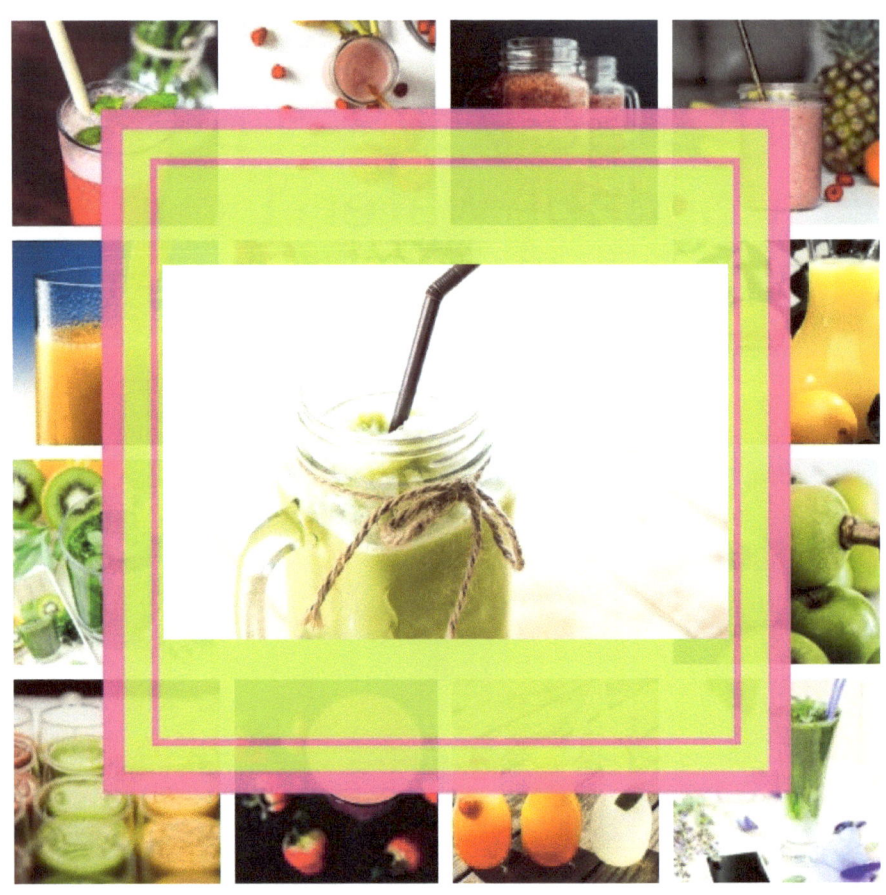

Green grapes 4-5
Coconut milk 1 small cup
Spinach 1 cup

It feels health and fit now!

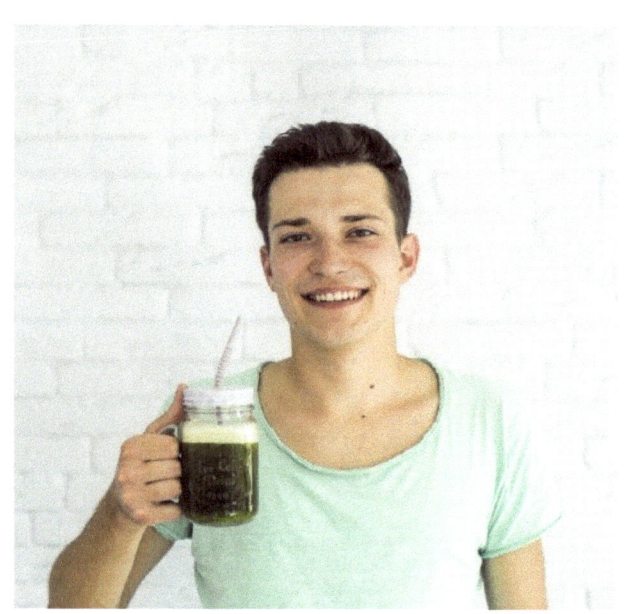

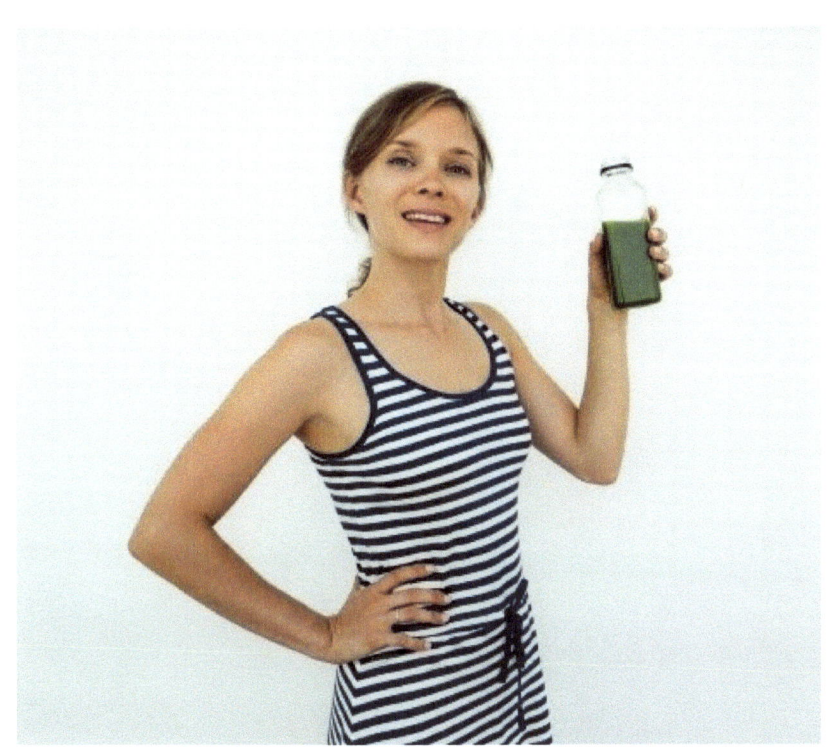

Want More Enjoyable Books?
Just Visit

www.ingramcontent.com/pod-product-compliance
Lightning Source LLC
Chambersburg PA
CBHW060821290526

45792CB00005BB/1754

9 781093 316353